Bad Habits and Good Habits:

How to Stay Healthy, Beautiful, and Young

TABLE OF CONTENTS

INTRODUCTION

Our culture is overly obsessed with health and beauty, and for no small reason. Working hard to stay healthy and live longer is a noble pursuit. Those who follow this kind of life usually look better than those who don't when they're 60; plus, they tend to live longer. This is the reason why celebrities don't seem to age, at least those who take good and proactive care of their health.

Pursuing a healthy life is great, but it's usually not that easy. Finding reliable information can be difficult, especially in this digital era. The data is one click away from you; but there's so much of it, it can become confusing. By the end, you don't know who to trust.

If you're reading this book, congratulations! You've found a reliable, science-based guide about healthy habits. Leading a healthier lifestyle isn't as hard as it seems. We're going to focus on identifying the patterns that will make sure you get healthy. We're also going to work on the easiest way to accomplish them.

With no further ado, let's change our lives for the better!

CHAPTER 1:

Reasons To Protect Your Health

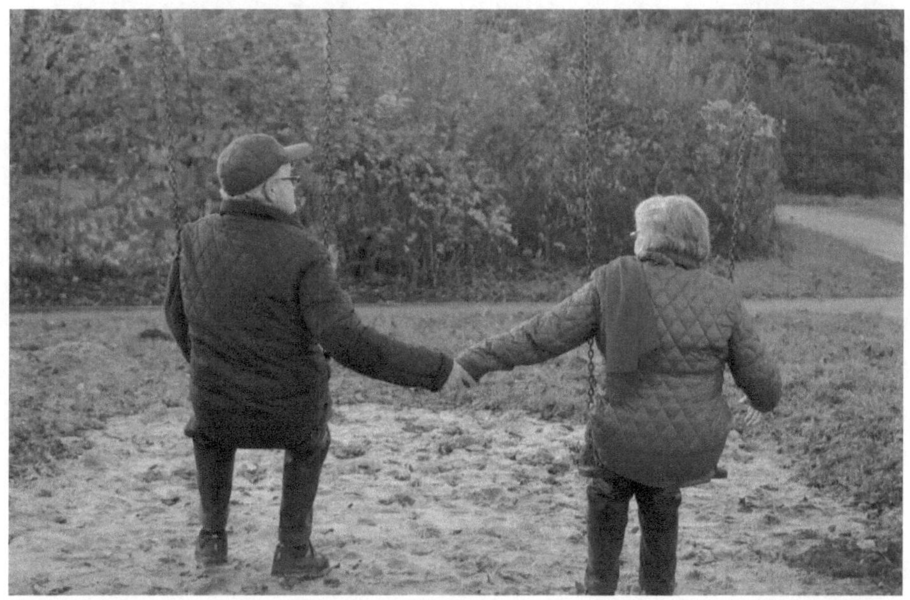

As you're reading this, the chances are that you already have an idea about why should you improve your health. The path to a healthier lifestyle is not impossible to travel, but it's long, and it may get hard. It's essential to keep your focus on the reasons why you are willing to do this. When you think about all you have to gain, it's absolutely worth it!

Saving money

Depending on where you live, healthcare can get expensive. In the year 2017, workers in the USA paid about 4,500$ to 8,300$ on average in healthcare[1]. Even if you live in a country with a national healthcare system, sickness still represents a cost to you and your family. People in these countries are often required to pay for some services or find themselves in need to solve their situations in the private sector due to inefficiency in the public health service.

Avoid unemployment

Chronic illness is bad for business. If you're self-employed, there's simply no way for you to produce money if you're seriously sick. If you work as an employee, they surely won't be glad to be left without you for an extended period. In some countries, such as in the USA, some laws[2] act in these cases. These regulations, however, often do not guarantee payment during your time of absence. Risking your health isn't a smart financial move. Apart from the medical bill, you risk losing your job.

Live longer

Young and relatively healthy people often do not care about their health. We all start caring once we reach old age and begin hearing the clock ticking. Health must never be taken for granted since the lack of it can considerably shorten your life expectancy. It comes as no surprise for anyone that leading a healthy life has been proved to raise your life expectancy[3]. This may not seem important when you're young, but trust me, as you get older, you'll see how short life is. Then, you'll wish you had more time.

Be the best version you can be for your loved ones.

Habits are first created in the family core. The American diet is passed on from generation after generation. It's specifically taught by the parents and perpetuated by the sons. If your children are barely ten or twelve years old and you're starting to feel the way your body is not the way it used to be, you know you didn't live with healthy habits. As a result, the only way to make sure that your kids are going to be healthier than you are is to set an example. Only by achieving healthy habits will you be able to pass them onto your offspring.

Keep your mind sharp

Crosswords and Sudokus are great for avoiding any form of dementia, but shielding your mind from Alzheimer doesn't stop there. Some studies prove that a healthy diet, rich with antioxidants, is also related to a lower risk of developing the disease[45]. Living over 80 years is no good if you start forgetting your surroundings by the age of 60. Some consider oblivion a worse fate than death. Nonetheless, there's no need to be afraid. It's possible to save your mind through healthy habits.

Avoid the nursing home.

There are two types of grandparents. Some grandparents seem as strong as an oak, live by themselves, and are even able to care for their grandchildren and have fun with them. Some others, on the contrary, need to be taken care of proactively. These older people cannot be trusted with kids' safety due to adults' current health or poor autonomy. Some grandparents end up living with one of their children, often feeling like a burden to their family. In the worst cases, they end in nursing homes. The difference between these types of grandparents is that the first ones led a healthier lifestyle than the last ones. Being able to enjoy your freedom and autonomy during your golden years requires work, but it's worth it.

Improve your mental health

We live in an era of mental health awareness. We are all sure that mental health is vital for happiness, work productivity, and even physical health. There are cultures, as well as some fields of work, that are especially prone to developing stress and anxiety. Nutrition[6] plays an essential role in managing anxiety. The same can be said about striving to have good sleep hygiene and doing exercise. Eating a balanced diet also helps reduce the symptoms of depression[7]. Mind and body are the same. Mental health and physical health are correlated.

There's much to gain from a healthy lifestyle and a lot to lose if we live in wrong way. Keep this in mind as you start your journey towards developing healthy habits.

CHAPTER II:

Illness, Aging, and Dying

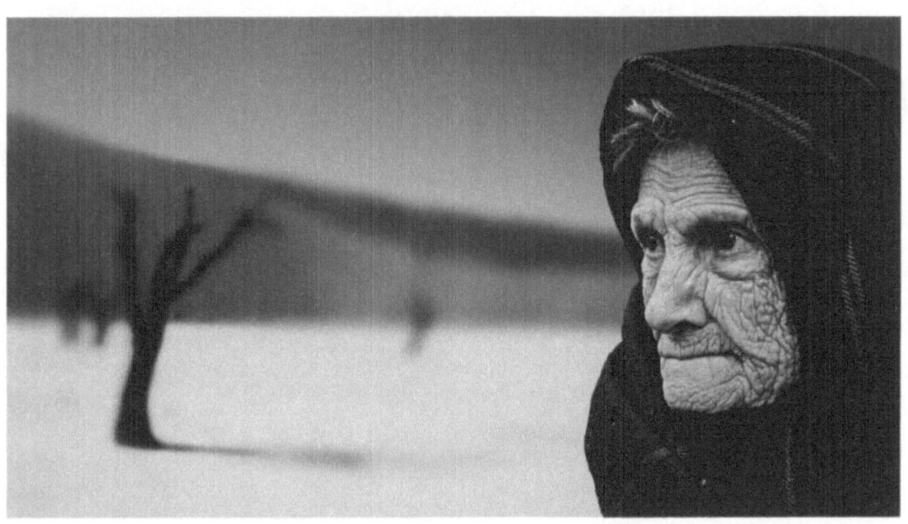

Let's break down one pair of myths regarding the health process before we start working on what will truly make us healthy.

What kills a person: Old age or disease?

Our bodies don't come with a timer ready to sound off and take us away. When people say that someone "died of old age," they don't mean it literally. Nobody dies of old age[8]. We all perish from an underlying cause. Most of us perceive this as the unavoidable consequence of coming to a certain age. It may convenient to think about it that way, that may rid us of responsibility, but the truth is that we die due to the consequences of the way we lived.

Indeed, our organs don't work as well as they used to when we're old, but that's no excuse for not taking care of them. Acquiring healthy habits that will make us live longer is our responsibility. Our bodies are more agile if we exercise. Our blood pressure is more vigorous, and we risk fewer heart diseases if we keep an active life. Food is the deciding factor. A healthy diet will save us from heart conditions[9], reduce the risk of cancer[10], diabetes mellitus, while even lowering its progression[11], and improve our chances regarding renal diseases[12]. These are all the leading causes of death, especially at old age, and they're all preventable.

Our hands aren't tied either in regards to cellular damage and ageing. A diet rich in antioxidants is also related to cellular preservation[13]. Cellular damage and ageing is the closest thing we have to a "lifeforce hourglass". Inevitably, 'we'll all get wrinkles at some point in our lives (unless of course, we die at a young age), but it's possible to delay them. A healthy diet, drinking enough water and avoiding bad habits that damage our body are all ways to preserve our cellular regeneration and slow the aging process.

The concept of "dying of natural causes" rids us of the responsibility of looking after ourselves and our health. To take these recommendations seriously, we must change that mindset.

What Causes Disease?

Health is conceived as a balance between the person and its surroundings by the UN. In this sense, we're used to thinking that being healthy is just not being sick, which is looking at things the other way around. Health is balance and equilibrium. We must actively work on remaining healthy instead of just avoiding being ill. Thinking this way makes us worry about our health only when the first symptoms of illness start to show. We have to understand that sickness is something that appears when we are careless about our health. Diseases appear when we lack health: that's the right way to look at it.

The concept of the epidemiologic triangle illustrates this very well. Sickness comes from the interaction between a susceptible host, an external agent, and environmental factors. It isn't as simple and straightforward as we usually perceive it. The pathogenesis process is complicated, especially in chronic diseases, which take our lives. Conditions such as hypertension, cancer, diabetes mellitus, kidney failure, heart attacks, and strokes, are all the result of the interaction between many factors. There's often a genetic component, of course; we can't control it, but thankfully it doesn't make a significant difference concerning our lifestyle choices[14]. Diseases, especially chronical diseases, potentially lethal diseases, are multifactorial. In this manner, we may look at the risk factors that develop diseases as something to avoid; and in essence, that's right. But, a better way to put it would be that, to prevent illness, we must aim for healthier habits. By pursuing health, instead of avoiding disease, we switch our gaze and start working on the offence. This puts us on the right mindset to make changes in our life that are meant to stay. To stay healthy, live longer, and have a better experience, we must create healthy habits that will last for a lifetime.

CHAPTER III:

How to Embark on the Right Path

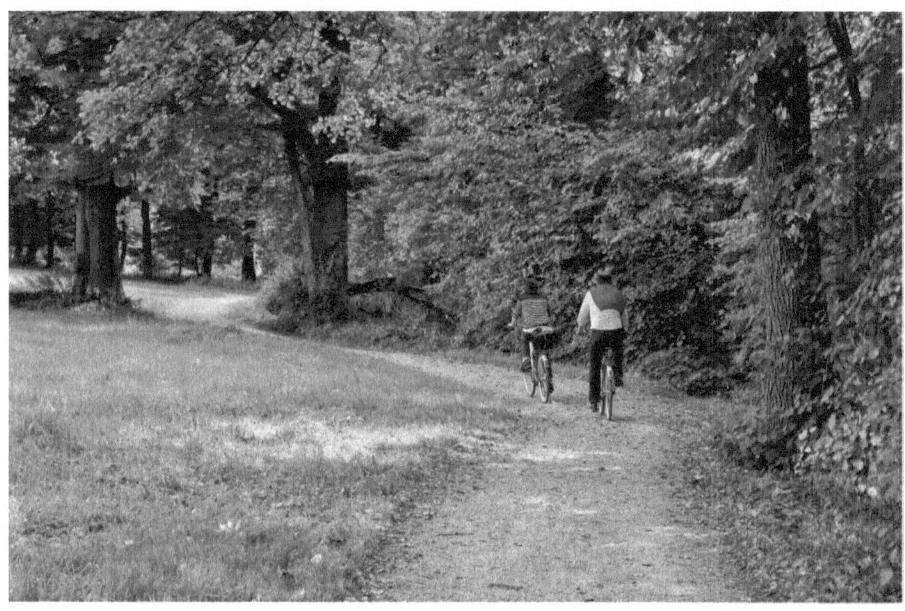

So, we already know that being healthy is hugely desirable. There aren't many things in this world that beat being healthy and living longer, and they certainly aren't bacon, chips, or cigarettes. You're now willing to start walking the path towards a healthier life, but in this era of information and confusion, the question remains, where to start?

Recognize the Facts

We can't walk this path without making some sacrifices. It's as simple as that. If you're one of those people who are used to drinking every weekend, having a bag of Cheetos whenever you feel the need to, and feel utterly displeased by the idea of exercising, you must understand that you need to make some changes. I'm not going to sugarcoat this for you. This is going to be hard. We're going to find a way to make it as easy as it may be, but it's still going to be very difficult. You didn't come here looking for an easy way out. There are no easy, long-term, realistic ways to stay healthy. Our culture's got us used to normalize healthy habits, especially if you live on the western side of the world. Plus, if you've tried other schemes that promise an easy path, you've probably failed, so you should already perceive that as the wrong way to go.

This is going to take willpower. You'll probably benefit greatly from the help and support from your family and friends, maybe even need it. You're going to make severe changes in your life, and this is the only way to improve and be healthy.

Have Common Sense

This may be hard for some of us, primarily since we're taught, counterintuitively, that some bad habits are not as bad as they seem. They are indeed, and before I show you evidence that tells you why, I'll advise you to trust in your common sense. You probably don't need anyone to tell you that overeating sugar or fats are bad for you. You already know that a diet based on KFC and coke isn't beneficial for you. Alcohol may be fun, but it's highly detrimental to your health. You don't need to see evidence to know that drinking is harmful to you. Smoking is one of the worst habits you could have. It's terrible for your wallet. It's catastrophic to your health and well-being, and there is no way to stay healthy while maintaining a smoking habit[15]. Of course, you don't need someone to tell you that stronger drugs are harmful to you. If you're always tired and you know that you don't sleep enough, you probably know what to do to fix that situation. Plus, being still on a bad mood is also bad for your mental and physical health, and if you're not sure how could it affect your physical health, you're still very aware that it isn't suitable for you.

Your common sense already tells you that you need to exercise to stay healthy and that you should eat enough vegetables to get all the nutrients that your body requires. You must drink enough water because hydration is essential. You must get enough sleep, and you should care for your mental health and well-being. Common sense is a useful compass whenever you're in doubt. The most important thing is to trust your instincts instead of following the bad habits perpetuated by your culture, especially when some part of you believes that they're not right for you.

Change Your Habits

Our everyday actions build our behaviors. These daily actions, these choices we make day after day, are all a consequence of our habits. Habits may be perceived as the core of our behaviors. They're like a machine that produces the pieces of our daily puzzle. If we teach those machines that we must wake up at 5:00 am every single day to do a mild routine of exercise, once it's configured that way, doing so will come as naturally to us as

Sleep habits are the key to changing our lives. That's where we'd like to start when we aim to live in a healthier way.

You are what you eat: Why does our health depend on food?

Our diet is the cornerstone of being healthy. A healthy diet is more efficient in keeping us healthy than working out in, for example, avoiding cancer[16] [17]. The most efficient way, not to say the only efficient way, to reduce our LDL cholesterol levels is through a healthy diet[18]. LDL cholesterol is a ruling factor in the development of atherosclerosis, which produces angina and heart attacks. This is a process that is developed since our childhood[19], and it's mostly due to the predominance of an unhealthy diet. The American Heart Association even recognizes the importance of a dietary approach to reduce high blood pressure, the DASH diet[20]. This nutritional focus recommends weight loss, consuming less salt, less saturated fats and cholesterol, alcohol, and more potassium, low-fat dairy products, fruits, and vegetables. The DASH diet may even prove to be essential for protecting diabetic patients from the effects of high blood pressure[21]. Herbs, berries, fruits, nuts, and other vegetal products give us the most top supply of antioxidants[22], which are vital for reducing oxidative stress-related diseases such as cancer, also cell damage and ageing. Some of this evidence inclines us to think that a healthy diet is even more vital than medication, which is the case in some studies regarding metabolic acidosis and kidney failure[23].

The evidence is right there in case you need to see for yourself. Every responsible internist focuses significantly on health. In the early stages of Diabetes Mellitus type 2, the treatment focuses on a healthy diet. If that much is achieved, there's no need to receive pharmaceutical treatment. Your diet should be low on saturated fats, salt, processed sugar, and LDL cholesterol. This means no candies, snacks, fried food, and reducing meat. Your diet should also be rich in fruits, vegetables, and other vegetal products. You will benefit from replacing meat products for vegetal products, and avoiding fat products at all costs. Your diet should be planned. Now that you have a general idea of what it must look like, you need to start buying your groceries differently. Think of your refrigerator as the most reliable reflection of your current health status. Is it full of beers, cold pizza, and pork chops ready for dinner? That's not right for you and you know it. Is your refrigerator full of colorful vegetables? Do you have small pouches of peanuts or fruit cups waiting for you if you feel hungry between meals? That's the way it should be. That's the only way you'll manage to stay healthy.

CHAPTER IV:

Everything You Need To Know About Healthy Eating

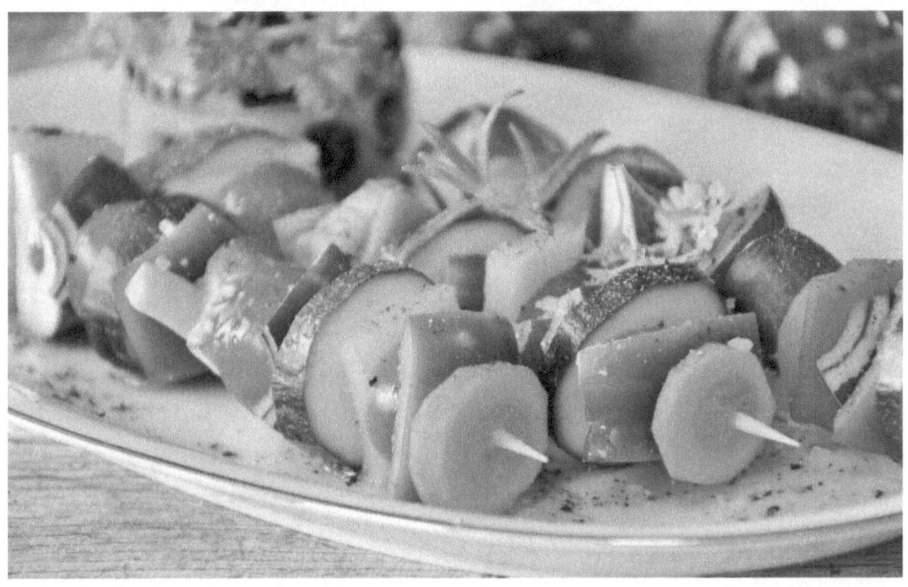

You should be already convinced of the benefits of following a healthy diet. You now have a broad idea of what to get next time you go to the supermarket and why. Now, let's get down to business!

The diet trap

If you want to follow a diet, first of all, you must stop thinking about it as such. We perceive foods as temporary solutions to our problems. They've been sold to us as something that you must follow rigorously for a couple of weeks, receive a benefit, and then go back to the way things were. If you were paying attention, you'd notice that this is not the case here. The changes you'll make here are meant to be permanent; it's the only way of staying healthy. People often try doing diets and fail because they're only thinking about all they're going to eat once it's finished. That's the diet trap; and if you're serious about being healthy, you won't fall for it.

Since this diet is not going to be temporary, there's no need to follow one of those "tuna and water" models. Your diet must be balanced; it has to contain animal and vegetal products, with a reasonable preference for fruits and vegetables. It must contain non-saturated fats, non-refined sugars, fibers, and proteins. Choosing wisely the food you take into your body will get you these nutrients while avoiding disease.

This doesn't mean that you should start eating like a rabbit right now. The changes you make must be gradual and realistic so that you'll be able to keep them in the long run. So try not to fall for that part of you that wants to be stunning the next time you have to wear a swimsuit. It'll come at its given time if you're constant, and more importantly, it'll persist.

It's All About The Math!

Losing weight if you're overweight, gaining it if you're underweight, or keeping it steady if you're healthy, it all comes down to the balance between caloric income and expense. There are many diets out there that speak about avoiding carbs or fats. They offer their reasons, but it can get somewhat confusing. Honestly, the only way to make sure you're going where you wish to go is by counting calories. It's not hard at all; we'll go through it step by step.

Your base caloric needs

Known as Basal Metabolic Rate, this is the daily number of calories your body needs for its primary functions. In sum, it refers to the number of calories you burn just for being alive. The Mifflin-St Jeor Formula is usually the preferred equation to calculate this[24]. It changes with biological gender, so let's start with women.

BMR = (4.536 × weight in pounds) + (15.88 × height in inches) − (5 × age) − 161

We'll illustrate this with an example, so let me introduce you, Amy. Amy is 37 years old, weighs 128 pounds, and stands 66 inches tall. In this case, the equation will go like this:

BMR = (4.536 × 128 pounds) + (15.88 × 66 inches) − (5 × 37 years old) − 161

BMR = 580.608 + 1048.08 − 185 − 161

BMR = 1282.688 calories

This could be rounded up to have a square number of 1283 calories.

The equation for men looks a little bit different.

BMR = (4.536 × weight in pounds) + (15.88 × height in inches) − (5 × age) + 5

We'll introduce you to Ralph for this example. Ralph is 42 years old, weights 168 pounds and stands 69 inches tall. His equation looks like this:

BMR = (4.536 × 168 pounds) + (15.88 × 69 inches) − (5 × 42 years old) + 5

BMR = 762.048 + 1095.72 − 210 + 5

BMR = 1652.768 calories

We could make this a square number and say 1653 calories as a BMR.

Daily caloric requirement

Your BMR would be enough for you if you didn't move at all. However, even if you're sedentary, there's still some activity that adds up for your caloric needs. To take this into account, we must multiply our BMR by a number that depends on our activity level. The equations look like this:

If you're sedentary, that is, little or no exercise, your DCR = BMR x 1.2

If you're lightly active, that is, exercising 1 to 3 days per week, your DCR = BMR x 1.375

If you're moderately active, that is, exercise 3 to 5 days per week, your DCR = BMR x 1.55

If you're very active, that is, exercise 6 or 7 days per week, your DCR = BMR x 1.725

And if you're super active, that is, tough exercise and a job that requires a high level of physical activity, your DCR = BMR x 1.9

So, to follow this example, if Amy went to the gym four times each week, and Ralph went jogging once per week, their daily calories requirement would look like this:

Amy's DCR = 1283 x 1.55 = 1988.65 calories

Ralph's DCR = 1653 x 1.375 = 2272.875 calories

If you've followed this process, you can write down your DCR. You're going to need it. Considering the western trend to be overweight, especially in America, you probably wish to lose weight. For this, you should subtract 500 calories from your DCR. If Amy, for example, wanted to lose weight, she would need to eat 1488.65 calories instead of 1988.65 calories. The same rule applies when you're aiming to gain weight, and you can keep your weight controlled by eating your DCR.

Get a kitchen scale

Now that you know how much calories you need to eat daily, you're likely wondering how to keep track of the calories you take to your mouth. Usually, you may see the energy (or caloric) value of packaged products. If you're having a cereal bar, a juice box, or even food at some fast-food restaurants, the nutritional value of what you're eating is readily available for you, so that you can count your calories with these products.

Things are different somehow when you want to eat mainly homemade food. Of course, since you are eating healthy, homemade food will be your primary source of nutrition. So you're probably wondering how to count calories in these situations. The best way to count calories is by using a kitchen scale. There are many tools available for you online once you look for calories per 100 grams of serving[25]. So, for example, cooked white rice gives you 94 calories per 100 grams of serving, 100 grams of grilled chicken breast gives you 157 calories, and so forth. Once you get used to this, by planning your meals and measuring your daily servings on a kitchen scale, keeping track of your calories is not hard at all. You can be in full control of what you eat, but if you consider that 100 grams of cooked chicken breast nets you 157 calories, but 100 grams of bacon nets you 882 calories, it's no wonder that keeping your weight down gets easier once you start choosing the right food to eat.

So, there you have it. From a numeric point of view, it's possible to control what you eat and your weight.

Fractional nutrition

There's a method to eat healthily, to care for your calories, and to avoid starving. Fractional nutrition is the idea that, instead of eating three big meals per day, we should have six meals. These meals should be 3 hours apart from each other and finish about 4 hours before we go to sleep. It may sound counterintuitive, but now that you know how to keep track of your calories, you can be sure to do this without overeating.

Fractional nutrition has its benefits; first of all, it gets rid of hunger. If you're one of those people who are always hungry, eating six planned meals a day is better than having a strict diet consisting of 3 meals, being hungry between meals, and eventually falling in the temptation of an unplanned snack. If your DCR is, for example, 1,800 calories, you can divide them in 3 bigger meals of 400 calories, and three meals of 200 calories each. You get your breakfast, lunch, dinner, and your snacks in-between without losing your focus or breaking your nutrition plan.

Eating more times per day also speeds up your metabolism. Have you ever seen somebody who's overweight and only eats two times per day? He or she usually has a late brunch and finishes one's days with a heavy dinner. It's no wonder that bodies work by turning the extra calories into fat deposits to have an energy backup for those long lapses of time without food. People with faster metabolisms usually eat more often, burn fat faster, and gain weight slower. Considering that those fats deposits are involved in the pathogenesis of diabetes[26], hypertension[27], and atherosclerosis[28], developing a faster metabolism is essential for your health.

Going back to those 2-meals overweight persons, if you obtain your most substantial meal before going to sleep, when are you supposed to burn those calories? Distributing your calories along your day allows you to burn those calories as you are consuming them.

Fractional nutrition is the healthiest way to eat. You should plan your meals, follow a schedule, and make sure that plan has enough fruits and vegetables, so you're treating your body the way it deserves.

Snacks are out of the question.

Your planned diet should always be enough to keep you satisfied. Nonetheless, if you're hungry because you're undereating to lose weight, you're anxious, or you have a craving, having a snack becomes challenging to avoid. A chocolate bar is around 190 calories, and a bag of chips is about 160. If the three smaller meals of your six planned meals consist of 150-200 calories, adding one of these is adding another full feed. It ruins your efforts, adds no nutritious value, and is loaded with processed sugar and saturated fats, which are bad for you.

If you're taking your health seriously, you're not thinking of snacks regularly. If you absolutely must have one, peanuts are the best kind of meal you could use. They are rich in protein, vegetable oils, and fibers, which we all should do an effort to integrate into our diets[29]. They're also great for mitigating hunger, so it's easy to have just a handful of them and feel full. It's not so hard to avoid snacks once you start applying the fractional nutrition diet correctly. For those times when you falter, make sure you protect your body while you do it.

Life is better when it's colorful.

As you plan your meals, you may find out that it's easier to have a full dish once you start adding vegetable portions. One hundred grams of chicken breast are already 157 calories, 100 grams of white rice are 96 calories, and 100 grams of raw tomatoes are 15 calories. This means that you can stick more than 600 grams of tomatoes instead of 100 grams of white rice and more than 900 grams of tomatoes instead of 100 grams of chicken breast. The lettuce is 11 calories; onions are 36, bell peppers are 26, and so on. Having a full dish is easier if you add a portion of salad. Half of your plate should be vegetables, according to The Dietary Guidelines for Americans[30].

Fruits and vegetables are high for your health[31]. They are rich in fiber, which is excellent for weight loss and for preventing heart diseases. They're also packed full of vitamins, minerals, and phytochemicals, which are also great for your health. These are all present in whole fruits and vegetables. You should have a full and colorful variety of them, always leaving the skin on to make sure you make the most of it.

Water is Life

The human body is 60% water[32]. It's vital for digestion, thermoregulation, blood pressure, tissue restoration, and renal function. It's also essential for our skin and hair, so if you're seeking a brighter, healthier, and younger skin, your solution comes in liquid form. The actual amount of water you should drink per day is controversial. Harvard[33] advises 2 or 3 cups of water per hour, others recommend drinking at least 85 ounces of water daily. Your main concern should be to drink water whenever you're feeling thirsty until you're satiated, make sure that it's no less than 50 ounces daily, and make sure it's plain water.

It's very accepted by our culture to substitute water with soft drinks. This isn't the healthiest choice since most soft drinks, such as soda, contain a high concentration of processed sugar and high caloric value. Soft drinks consumption is linked with poor dental health, overweight, diabetes, among other diseases. It's definitive that you should avoid soda at all costs. If you drink anything other than water, try having fruit and vegetable juice without sugar. You may add honey instead of white sugar, a complex and unrefined source of carbohydrates and minerals. There's nothing like a glass of fresh water to quench your thirst. Your mouth wants it, and your body is begging for it.

When should you eat protein?

First of all, almost every foodstuff has protein. When people speak about having protein in a meal, they're referring to having meat, chicken or any other ingredient with a substantial protein concentration. If you're a heavy lifter, you're well aware that your body needs protein to build muscular tissue, but how much is enough, and when should you have it?

Your body needs a minimum of 0.8 grams of protein per kilogram of body weight, which is 48 grams of meat per day if you weight 60 kilograms. This amount of protein should be raised to 1 gram per kilogram of bodyweight if you exercise lightly, 1.2 if you use moderately, and up to 1.6 grams per kilogram of bodyweight if you exercise heavily to restitute muscle tissue[34] This rule is simple enough, and it shows that you don't need as much protein as you probably thought you did, especially considering that a low protein diet is overall better for your health and for reducing the risk of cancer[35 36].

Now, as to when you should have it, you should definitively consume it during breakfast and lunch. It's harder for your body to digest protein, especially massive animal-sourced protein, so consuming it during dinner will result in having trouble to rest at night. Dinners should be focused on fruits and vegetables. Contrary to the American way, a vegetable broth is much better for you than a steak during dinner.

Cleansing your body

There's beauty in the concept of fasting days. Even if you're struggling to keep a healthy diet, your body is receiving toxins from animal-sourced foodstuff. It's highly recommended to place one of these fasting days at least twice a month. They'll help your body get rid of toxins, help with metabolism, and make you feel better. Fasting days should consist of no more than 25% of your CDR, or 500 calories for women and 600 for men[37], distributed solely between fruits and vegetables. You should drink lots of water, but also, having these 500 calories blended in green smoothies with kale, lemon, strawberries, and honey, is advisable. You could also benefit from apple slices to give your jaws some work and help you feel satiated. You'll start feeling better after these fasting days. Your body will be grateful, it'll also lift your spirit, and it's the best way to get rid of toxins clogging your body.

The healthier path

Here are seven of the most respected and famous experts in the science of nutrition. All of them promoted different diets.

John Tilden, Distinguished MD from Denver, exemplified an outstanding scientist who was historically deemed as one of the most skilled doctors. His methods of treatment included fasting and nutrition with a predominance of fruits and vegetables. He lived for more than 90 years and was actively engaged in therapy until the end of his life[38].

John Harvey Kellogg, MD was the director of the famous Battle Creek Sanatorium in Michigan.[39] He specialized in a vegetarian diet that helped restore health to many people. He was focused on preventive medicine, a health-aimed emphasis that would prevent the pathogenesis of illness.

Bernard McFadden was the writer of the famous 'Physical Culture Book' in 1901[40]. At first, he practiced vegetarianism but later settled on a mixed diet that included meat and fish. His food was more focused on bodybuilding. He was healthy and lived for almost 90 years.

St. Louis Estes was a pioneer and strict follower of a raw food diet during the late 20s and early 30s. Thanks to his diet, many patients regained their health[41].

Dr Benedict Lust was the founder of naturopathy in America in the first decade of the 20th century. He founded a large school of naturopathy in New York. Hundreds of followers spread his teachings throughout the world. Nowadays, naturopathy uses natural resources and diets to treat illnesses[42].

Dr. Henry Lindlahr founded the Lindlahr College of Natural Therapeutics during the first decade of the 20th century. He was the first to call for the return of therapy and prevention to natural methods. He was one of the first to call for the use of vitamin and mineral supplements[43].

Professor Arnold Ehret was one of the most excellent nutritionists. He created the "Mucus-Free Diet" treatment method, a solution to the existence of mucus in our diet, which he claimed to be the source of our diseases[44]. Many of his students reached full health in 80-90 years.

Even though they're researchers from the 20th century, they managed to achieve longevity, so they're worth referencing. Most of them promote natural vegan diets, which nowadays are backed with scientific research. Vegan diets are high for preventing anginas[45], cancer[46,47], diabetes[48,49], renal failure[50,51], and blood pressure[52,53,54]. This validates the point where populations that don't consume animal-sourced food are virtually free of heart conditions[55,56,57]. There's a benefit to be had over going vegan. It's scientifically proven to be healthier; it helps you reduce fats, cholesterol, lose weight, and make sure you get enough nutrients. There are never enough greens in your diet. Remember, there's no way for you to get different results if you keep living the way you were. To improve, you must change. After studying these famous experts, we have made a broad list of what to avoid and what should we replace food products; it encompasses the following:

- Refined sugar and products made from it, such as ice cream, jam, cakes, chewing gum, sugary drinks, pies, cookies, puddings, and artificial juices. It's better to have whole carbohydrates rather than processed sugars, so if you're ever in need of sweetening something, a spoonful of honey is significantly better than a teaspoon of white sugar.

- Ketchup, mustard, spicy tomato sauce, canned food. These are all products full of chemicals and preservatives that aren't good for your body.
- Salted foods: crisp, salted nuts, salted crackers, etc. Consuming salt is related to cardiovascular and renal diseases.
- Products made from peeled rice.
- Corn flakes and similar products.
- Fried foods represent a source of saturated fats, and they're heavily laden with useless calories.
- Saturated fatty and hydrogenated oils, including margarine.
- Alcohol, coffee, tea.
- Tobacco.
- Pork.
- Smoked products.
- Products that contain nitrates, such as ham, bacon, salami, and some other meat-related products.
- Flour products (white bread, cookies, cakes, waffles, pasta, spaghetti, pizza) are processed carbohydrates, which are deeply related to diabetes and often lack the vitamin, minerals, and nutrients that our bodies need.
- Stale vegetables.

In essence, eating healthier starts with knowing what to do, what to avoid, and how to plan your food to live longer.

CHAPTER V:

Start Moving!

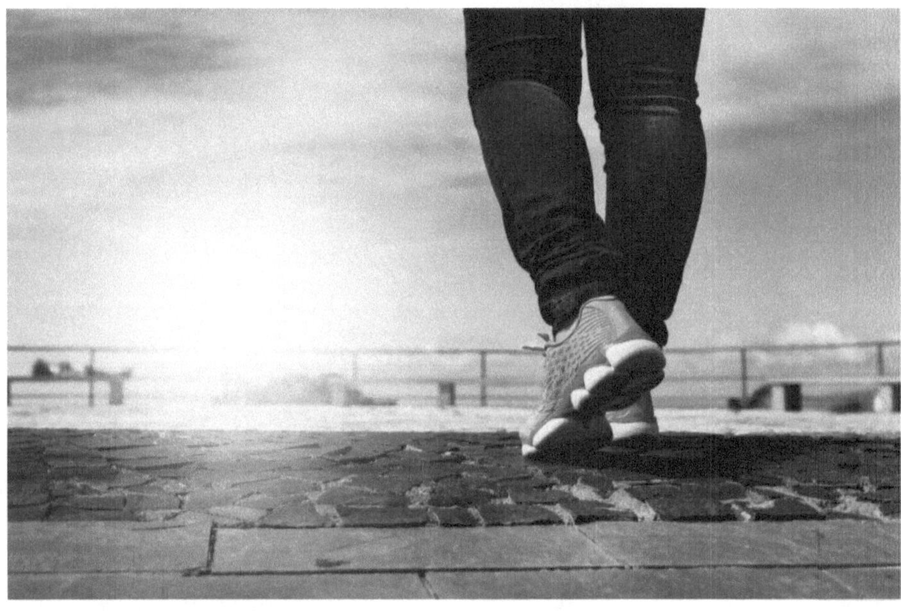

It's possible to be healthier just by having a healthy diet. It's viable to lose weight and keep it only by caring for what you eat. If you're one of those people who cannot stand the idea of doing exercise, you may believe that it's possible to skip this step, but the benefits that exercise bring to your life make a major difference. Physical activity protects us from the development of cardiovascular diseases, cancer, diabetes, hypertension, obesity, depression, and osteoporosis[58]. The more physical activity you integrate into your life, the less probability you face of developing one of these diseases. People who exercise tend to be happier and people are more comfortable when they're physically active[59]. This is a result of feeling physically better, as well as having your body release endorphins[60], which are directly related to feeling pleasure.

If one of the reasons why you want to lose weight and be healthier is looking better, you should prioritize exercise. The relation between the calories you eat and the calories you burn dictate whether you're gaining, losing, or staying in your current weight. Training dictates the way your body is going to earn, lose, or keep that weight. If you want to get rid of your flabby arms and a pot belly, there's no other way to do it than exercising. Losing weight only makes your body a smaller and lighter version of what it is, it's up to you to build your body the way you want it to look.

How much exercise is enough?

Each week you should do at least 150 minutes of moderate aerobics or 75 minutes of intense aerobics[61]. Moderate aerobics could be brisk walking, jogging lightly, or swimming. Intense aerobics could be playing sports such as tennis or basketball, running, or aerobic classes. You should also do some strength training at least twice per week. The major muscle groups you should exercise are legs, chest, back, and abs. You could work them all together in activities such as rock climbing, or individualize them in the gym. The health benefit is more significant if you manage to double the weekly amount of aerobics. This means 30 daily minutes of aerobic activity, so starting each day with a jog is highly advisable. Also, if you're a very busy person, high-intensity programs such as high-intensity interval training manage to fit short and efficient training routines. Exercising in the morning is the best way to start your day, followed by a nutritious breakfast.

Starting to exercise

If you're a complete beginner, you may make mistakes while starting to work out. Here's what you should look out for:

An efficient training routine should always have you sweating. If you're walking so slow that you don't force your body, you may as well be sitting on your couch.

Breathing, drinking water, and looking out for your vital signs is very important. For this matter, it's helpful to have a smartwatch to track your fitness and vitals.

Looking after your posture is very important if you don't want to injure yourself during your workouts. You must always keep your back straight, try to move in circular motions, and practice the technique of your strength exercises before doing them.

Wait for an hour after eating before you exercise. Exercising in the morning before breakfast is ideal; however, but if time isn't possible, you should never start right after you've eaten. Also, having food after your exercise routine is perfect, especially after your strength training. In turn, your body can start the process of rebuilding your muscle tissue.

Don't be discouraged if you're unable to do as much exercise as you initially intended. If you get tired in the middle of your running session, you can always catch a breath for five minutes and go back to it. Anything is better than avoiding exercise, and as you get better, you'll start to see it's becoming easier for you.

CHAPTER VI:

Stop alcohol and smoking

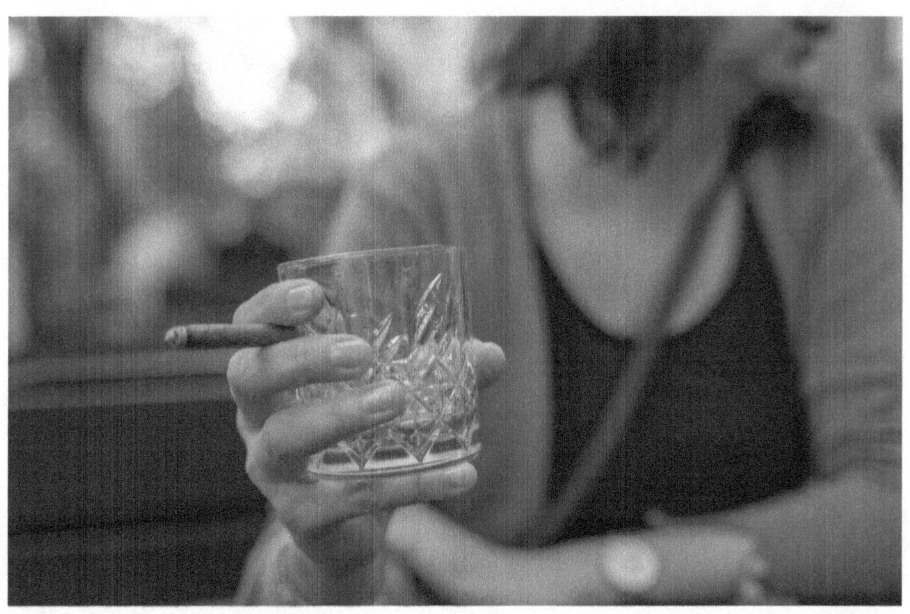

Bad habits are an eminent part of our culture. We see happy people drinking, smoking and doing drugs every day in the media. As we become conscious of the damage from these habits to our health, we can curb the consumption of these products. Yet, there are many people still poisoning their bodies with these toxins, especially alcohol consumers, since many people consider it normal to drink every weekend.

Is beer that bad?

Having just a couple of drinks every weekend is socially acceptable. It's often criticized to avoid all alcoholic beverages, even though consuming them is detrimental to human health. The truth is that even the slightest consumption of alcohol is directly related to cardiovascular diseases, cancer, disability, and the overall deterioration of health[62]. If you're taking your health seriously and you stop having soda, for example, it's absurd even to consider having a beer. This becomes more serious once you think that one bottle of beer contains 140 to 180 calories, so having one or two beers gives you the number of calories provided by a whole meal, without the nutritional value.

Is it hard for you to abstain from alcohol for good? Ask yourself the following questions:

- Have you ever felt you should cut down your drinking?

- Have people annoyed you by criticizing your drinking?

- Have you ever felt bad or guilty about your drinking?

- Have you ever had a drink first thing in the morning to steady your nerves or get rid of a hangover (eye-opener)?

These questions come from the CAGE questionnaire[63]. If you answer two or more of these questions affirmatively, there's a chance you have a drinking problem, so you should further investigate this with a professional. The right professionals seek are clinical psychologists, psychiatrists, and therapists.

Leaving alcohol out of your life should be an absolute choice if you want to improve your health. There's no way to be completely healthy if you consume even the slightest amount of alcohol.

Is there any way to be healthy and smoke?

No, there isn't. Smoking is one of the most harmful habits you could take for your health[64] [65]. It's related to cancer, lung disease, heart disease, multi-organic disease, and even mental disease. More than a bad habit, it's an addiction. Most smokers do it because they started at a very young age when they were unconscious and reckless, and now they're unable to stop.

Stopping alcohol consumption may be more complicated than quitting burgers, especially if you've been smoking for more than a couple of years. Still, it's a step everyone should make, even if you're not aiming to maximize your health. People often fail because they do it by themselves. They treat this as if it were a matter of willpower, and to a certain degree, it truly is. Still, the physiological need of your body for tobacco is so strong that sometimes it becomes almost impossible to tackle this problem with sheer willpower. You should always seek professional help and support from your family and close ones when you want to quit smoking. Some methods and therapies such as hypnosis have shown great results[66]. It's possible to quit smoking, which is imperative to your health; on the contrary, it's just a matter of knowing how to do it.

I'm in deep trouble

Being addicted to other drugs such as cannabis, ecstasy, cocaine, and heroin is death sentence when it comes to being healthy. These drugs have an adverse impact on your life. They're also related to mental health and neurological health issues, as well as cardiovascular diseases. Here is where you should start in your quest for health if you're currently addicted to one of these substances. Much like with cigarettes, stopping the consumption of these drugs takes professional health. In this case, it's urgent to consult a psychiatrist or medical professional as quickly as you can to start your path of recovery.

CHAPTER VII:

Healthy Body, Mind, and Soul

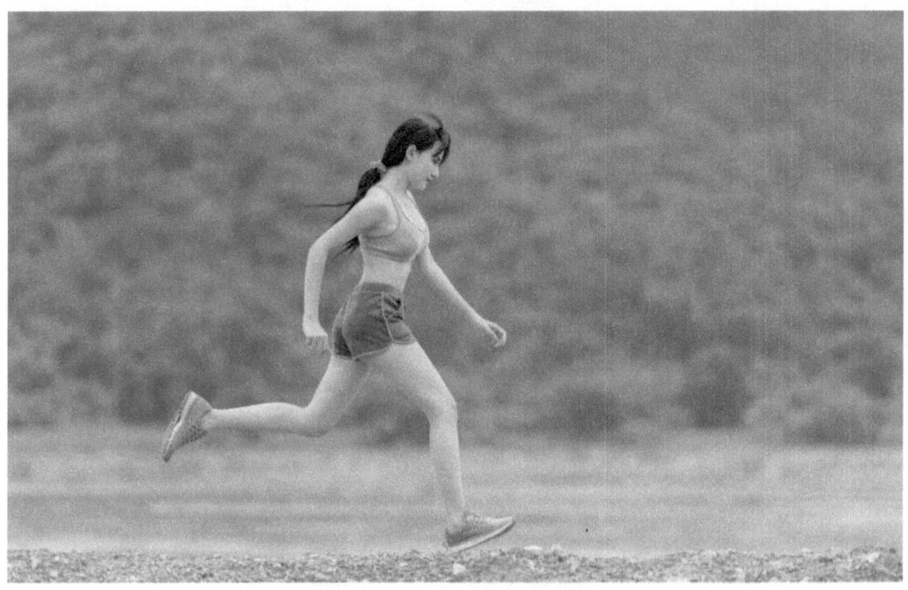

Being healthy isn't only a matter of eating and exercising. In reality, the job is not complete if you don't take care of your mental health. There's a strong correlation between mental health and physical health[67]. The three conditions essential for your health in conjunction with a healthy diet, physical exercise, and spiritual balance.

Stress management

A small amount of stress is unavoidable. Stress is an adaptative response of our body, and it's present in our daily lives. When the amount of stress becomes chronic and our coping mechanisms fail, stress becomes a disease bearer[68][69]. If you feel like you're always in a rush, anxiety is eating at you, here's what you ought to do to manage your stress properly.

You should, by all means, stop consuming caffeine. Coffee and energy drinks increase our amount of stress, as such, removing them from your life is the right choice.

Let go of the wheel. Understanding that you're not in full control of everything that's going on around you is crucial to your stress management.

If you feel like you're going too fast, take a pause. Nothing is more important than your health. Taking time for yourself, breathing deeply, appreciating the beauty of your surroundings, and doing something you love: these are all great for stress management before you go back to your work.

Make sure that your daily activities aren't bursting with work. It's advisable to follow the time blocking method, plan your days to make the most of your time and make sure to make time for relaxation.

Avoid taking responsibilities that you don't have the time to. Once you're able to plan your daily activities, you'll know when you have the space for a new project, and when you don't.

Make sure to eat healthily, exercise regularly, and sleep properly. These are all very important for stress management as they shield us from the chronic adverse effects of stress.

Inadequate coping mechanisms and habits are often related to stress. Avoid substance abuse and bingeing to cope with stress. Instead, you should rely on socializing with your close ones and making time for yourself.

Stress is a common disease in our current society, but it doesn't need to be that way. Healthily managing stress is possible.

Beauty sleep

Poor sleep habits and sleep disruption are related to mental disease, hypertension, diabetes mellitus, metabolic syndrome, weight issues, and cancer[70]. Ideally, you should sleep for 8 hours straight. The number of hours you sleep is not the only thing that matters. It's essential to make sure that you're sleeping properly. If you're often waking up in the middle of the night, or you wake up after a long night of sleep, and you don't feel well-rested, here's what you should do to improve your sleep habits:

Your bed should be intended for rest and pleasure. Working, studying, or even watching television in your bed will make you connect it mentally to stressful situations. This makes it harder for you to sleep and rest properly on your bed. Your bed should remain a sacred place; thus, the only activities you're supposed to do in your bed are lovemaking, resting, and sleeping.

Get away from all screens at least one hour before sleeping! This time should be used for reading, thinking about your day and drawing conclusions out of it. Your last meal should be at least 3 hours before you sleep to ensure your body isn't burdened with the task of digesting your last meal while you're trying to sleep.

Avoid caffeine and stimulating substances. These should also be avoided for health reasons, so they shouldn't have a place in your life as things are right now.

Making sure that you sleep enough is essential for your stress, health, and overall happiness. Make sure that you're not losing your valuable sleep, or wasting it by sleeping poorly.

Cultivate your soul

As you plan your day, be sure that you leave time for yourself and the things you love. No one can truly function like a machine. If we wish to lead a healthy life, it must also be a happy life. Making time for yourself isn't difficult. Your biggest guide will be yourself. As you do something that you like, take a moment to step out of it and see it from an outside perspective. If you're genuinely having fun and enjoying yourself, this is an activity that you must continue doing. If instead, this activity is more of an obligation, and you don't feel good doing it, stop. There are too many obligations in our life to make leisure time one of them.

CHAPTER VIII:

Why Aren't We Healthy Yet?

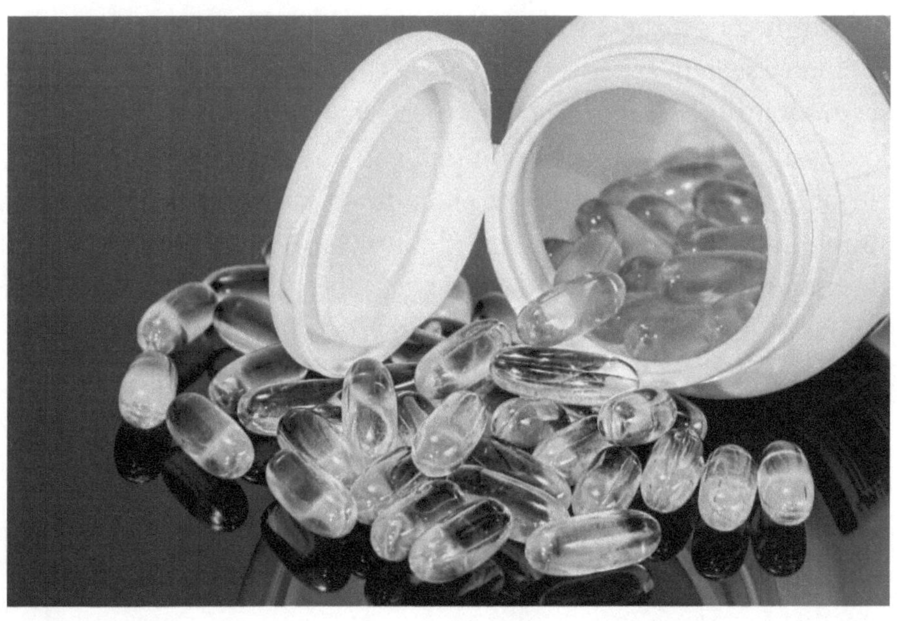

The Internet will give tens of thousands of books if you enter the word "health" in the search box. Humanity has never had such a wealth of information on how to lose weight, how to maintain health, and how to gain longevity. There have never been so many books, videos, seminars, clubs, gyms, and other opportunities to be a healthy person. We have the opportunity to choose the healthy and delicious food that we wish. We have one of the best levels of medical care in the world. Until the middle of the 20th century, our predecessors did not have such an opportunity. A logical and fair question arises. Why do we care about overweight, health and life expectancy, if all the resources we need are right there? Why are we still unable to be healthy if we have all of this at our disposal?

The answer lies in the quality of the information. In this era of information, there are tons of people selling secure solutions to our health problems. We often see natural diets that promise to make us healthy in just a couple of weeks. Pills, supplements, and products that promise they'll change our bodies and make us healthier overnight flood the Internet and media. The hard truth, as you should've seen in the early chapters of this book, is that there are no secure solutions. Being healthier means changing your lifestyle. To lose weight, stay young, live longer, and stay healthy, you must get rid of your bad habits and produce new, healthier ones. It's that simple, and it is as accurate right now as it was hundreds and thousands of years ago. The ways to achieve health, beauty, and longevity have not changed, and now, we have scientific studies that prove it.

We may not be healthy right now, especially if we follow these easy-out plans advertised online. Scientific studies should always back your take on achieving health and endured the proof of time. That's the only way to make sure that all your hard work won't be in vain.

CHAPTER IX:

Where Do We Start? The Role of Habits in Our Lives

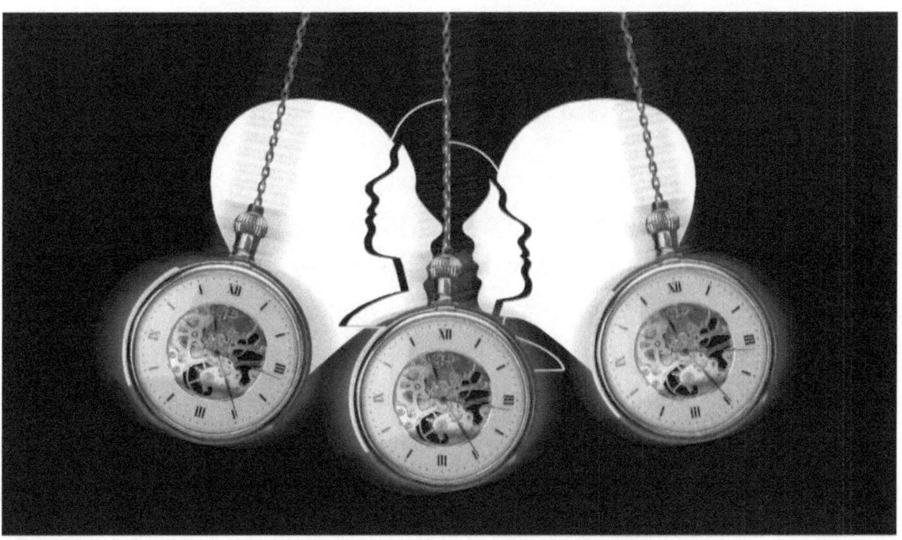

Aristotle stated that virtue comes from repetition. He stated "We are what we repeatedly do. Excellence, then, is not an act, but a habit". One could only be virtuous if our good deeds happened often. That's the core of healthy habits. As much as it's true that we're unhealthy for our bad habits, we'll only be truly healthy once we create good habits. Since the pursuit of health isn't something we can turn on and off, but an ongoing and lasting battle, the only way to be healthy is to create long-lasting changes in our life. Accordingly, that's where habits play a major role.

We can form new habits that will rule our behaviors for the rest of our lives. We can plan them as if we were configuring the changes in a machine. We must look at the lives we're leading right now, compare them with the healthy lives we want to live, count the differences between them, divide them in new habits, and start working in them one by one. This way, we can create the process of metamorphosis that'll change our lives for the better. Choosing to exercise, for example, is a goal that, once it's turned into a habit, will come automatically to us. Some say that it only takes 21 days to make a new habit, science states that after ten weeks[71], all patterns will be automatic. This is our Success Plan for Health. Without this, all the advice of the world will be useless. The key is to focus on the habits of a healthy person. Your brain is rebuilding.

You'll begin to live like a healthy person. Stop believing in easy and short solutions. There's no way to improve your health and lose weight in three days without doing anything. If you're looking for Health Formulas, they've been here since the beginning of our existence. At the beginning of humankind, there were no formulas or professors. We had simple and healthy food, exercise, and no alcohol and tobacco. Back then, we were healthy, and the problem of weight loss didn't exist. Now, we must learn to live bit by bit healthily. Becoming healthy is a process that may take six months, a year, or even a little bit more. It doesn't matter; every step up the ladder will make you feel better, more powerful, and healthier. Once you get one good habit, you'll feel much stronger. And you'll succeed because you're doing things the right way.

The strategy of mini-habits in eating and maintaining health

So now we know everything about what's healthy, and what isn't. We've obtained a picture of what our healthy life will look like, and we've planned the habits we'll work on to achieve this. Some practices, we will need to tackle entirely, such as smoking. The only way to quit smoking is to stop smoking entirely. We can't reduce smoking bit by bit until it's out of our lives: that doesn't work. Now, this doesn't apply to the rest of the changes we could make in our lives. If you're finding it hard to tackle these new habits, such as a healthy diet, for example, there's a more natural and more effective way to win this battle.

Mini habits are smaller, more achievable, versions of our complete patterns. If willpower is your weak point, you may find that it's easier for you to drop all sodas before you lose all refined sugars from your diet, for example. Doing something, no matter how small, is preferable to doing nothing. It's also more comfortable, safer, and will work just as excellent in the long run. Let me give you an example, only to be sure everything is clear.

Your new diet should erase all saturated fats, processed sugars, count calories, reduce animal-sourced proteins, and increase vegetables and fruits. Instead of eliminating all processed sugar, you may divide this in mini habits such as no more bagged candy, no more homemade sweets and bakery, and no more soda and sugary soft drinks. Reducing fats could start with taking the pork out of your life, cutting out fatty snacks, eliminating fried food, and so on. Taking these small yet decisive steps is the way to win this battle and become healthier. There are several tenets you must know to understand and adequately apply this strategy.

- It's easier to form and secure easy habits than strict habits.

- Your inner motivations should drive your habits. This means that as much as we may want to create a reward system, the most effective way to create patterns is to be led by our reasoning.

- Track your progress to see your growth and feel motivated. It's easy to see where we fell, but not how much we've accomplished. Make sure to remind yourself day after day how strong and capable you are.

- New habits will get to be annoying at some point. That's alright, that means you're doing this the right way.

- Constancy is the breeding ground for habits. Your life and health will gain more from small daily changes than from significant changes made only once.

- Having a written list teaches your brain the relevance of its items. You should maintain a written record of the habits you'd want to have at any given point in your life.

- You'll know a behavior became a habit once it's easier to do it than to stop doing it. Once you do it without even thinking about it, after o your inner self knows so well that you'll do it no matter what that it stops worrying about it, and upon feeling excited about doing it, it becomes ordinary and boring.

That's the way to a healthy path. It's up to you to achieve it; the best part is that it all starts with one small and easy step.

CHAPTER X:

Some Recipes for Health Cooking

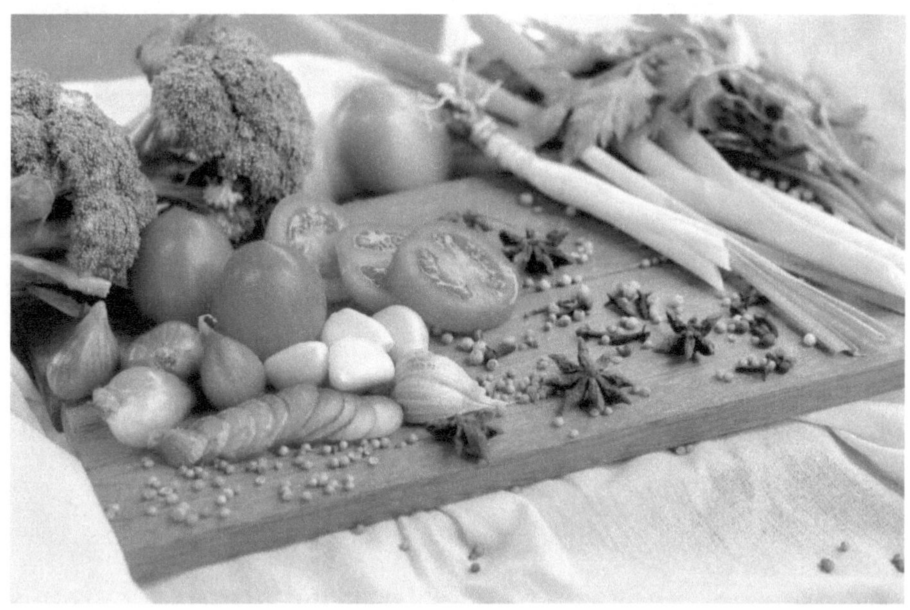

Here's an example of a meal plan for a day, based on 2,000 calories. It's based on a non-vegan diet by following the main principles of this book. This guide offers you an idea of what your planned meals should look like:

Non-Vegan Diet

Breakfast

A bowl of 100 grams of oat porridge and 30 grams of sliced strawberries, 400 calories.

Mid-day

A smoothie prepared with 250 grams of non-fat milk, 150 grams of no-fat yoghurt, 100 grams of bananas, 100 grams of strawberries, 50 grams of kelp, and one and a half teaspoons of honey, 300 calories.

Lunch

A dish of 120 grams of chicken breast, 100 grams of brown rice, and a green salad consisting of 50 grams of raw lettuce, 50 grams of fresh spinach, 50 grams of raw tomato, 50 grams of raw cucumber, 50 grams of cooked broccoli, dressed with 1 tablespoon of vinaigrette dressing, 420 calories. Try to use condiments over salt.

Mid-afternoon

A snack made with 50 grams of dried fruit and 20 grams of any mix of almonds, pistachios, cashews, or peanuts. The nuts may be roasted, and lightly salted is preferable. This encompasses 300 calories.

Dinner

A creamy soup with 50 grams of low-fat cream, 140 grams of potatoes, 100 grams of stir-fried onions, 50 grams of carrots, 50 grams of broccoli, and 100 grams of mushrooms. The onions should be stir-fried in olive oil. The baked potatoes, onions, carrots, and cream should be blended together. It's up to you to also mix in the broccoli or leave it whole, along with the slices of cooked mushrooms. This is 400 calories.

Last meal of the day

A fruit cup with 100 grams of Greek yogurt, 100 grams of sliced pineapple, 50 grams of red cherries, 50 grams of blue grapes, and 30 grams of strawberries. This is 180 calories.

CONCLUSION

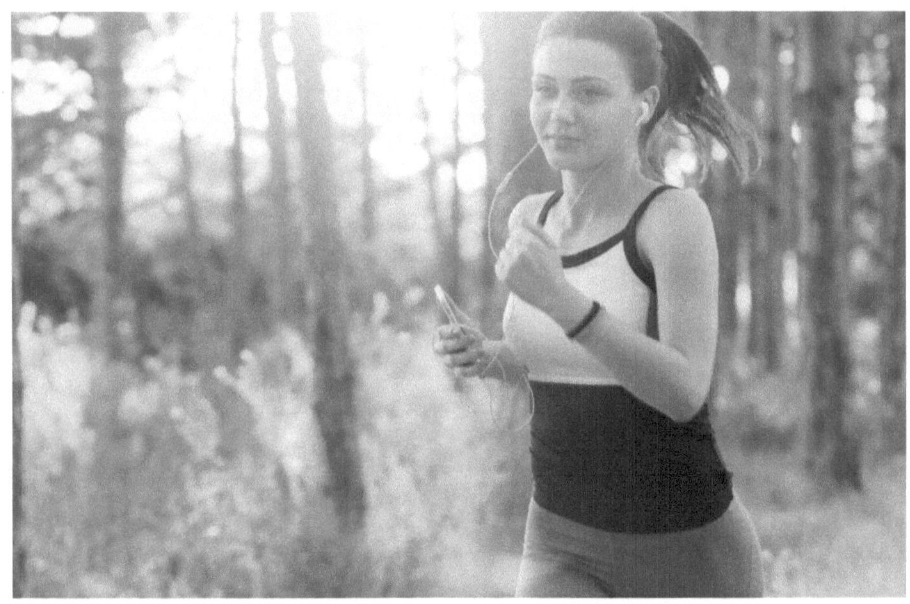

There's no easy path for health. Most bad habits are so normalized in our culture and the media that it may come as a shock to learn that we must drop them to become healthy. Plus, our minds will make this harder for us at the beginning. Some people will bring us support; some others make it more daunting for us. The road will often become challenging, but nothing will be in vain. The only thing that matters is to be sure of the path you're following. All your efforts will bring you profit and ensure that you live a longer life. The reason for this is that you've found a real, time-proofed, science-supported method in this book.

There's no easy path for health; there's only the right path. I'm sure you'll be able to see it through successfully.

BIBLIOGRAPHY

1. "Ranked: Cost of healthcare per capita in 21 different countries ...." March 7th 2019, https://www.businessinsider.com/cost-of-healthcare-countries-ranked-2019-3. Accessed on November 15th 2019.

2. "What Happens to Your Job if You Get a Terrible, Long-Term ...." September 10th 2018, https://melmagazine.com/en-us/story/what-happens-to-your-job-if-you-get-a-terrible-long-term-illness. Accessed on November 15th 2019.

3. "Impact of Healthy Lifestyle Factors on Life Expectancies in the ...." https://www.ahajournals.org/doi/full/10.1161/CIRCULATIONAHA.117.032047. Accessed on November 15th 2019.

4. "Impact of Healthy Lifestyle Factors on Life Expectancies in the ...." https://www.ahajournals.org/doi/full/10.1161/CIRCULATIONAHA.117.032047. Accessed on November 15th 2019.

5. "Journal of the American Geriatrics Society - Wiley Online Library." April. 27th 2015, https://onlinelibrary.wiley.com/doi/abs/10.1111/j.1532-5415.1997.tb01476.x. Accessed on November 15th 2019.

6. "Nutritional strategies to ease anxiety - Harvard Health Blog ...." August 29th 2019, https://www.health.harvard.edu/blog/nutritional-

strategies-to-ease-anxiety-201604139441. Accessed on November 15th 2019.

7. "Can Eating a Healthy Diet Really Help Treat Depression ...." October 9th 2019, https://www.livescience.com/changing-diet-helps-depression.html. Accessed on November 15th 2019.

8. "Natural Causes: What Does it Mean to "Die of Old Age?" February 6th 2014, https://www.aplaceformom.com/blog/2-6-2014-what-does-it-mean-to-die-of-old-age/. Accessed on November 15th 2019.

9. "A way to reverse CAD? - NCBI." https://www.ncbi.nlm.nih.gov/pubmed/25198208. Accessed on November 15th 2019.

10. "Effects of a low-fat, high-fiber diet and exercise ... - NCBI." https://www.ncbi.nlm.nih.gov/pubmed/16965238. Accessed on November 15th 2019.

11. "Effects of the High Carbohydrate-Low Calorie Diet ... - NCBI." https://www.ncbi.nlm.nih.gov/pubmed/20319961. Accessed on November 15th 2019.

12. "The Western-style diet: a major risk factor for impaired ... - NCBI." August 31st 2011, https://www.ncbi.nlm.nih.gov/pubmed/21880837. Accessed on November 15th 2019.

13. "The importance of antioxidant enzymes in cellular ... - NCBI." https://www.ncbi.nlm.nih.gov/pubmed/1450609. Accessed on November 15th 2019.

14. "Genes vs. Lifestyle: What Matters Most for Health? - WebMD." https://www.webmd.com/healthy-aging/features/genes-or-lifestyle. Accessed on November 15th 2019.

15. "The preventable causes of death in the United ... - NCBI - NIH." April 28th 2009, https://www.ncbi.nlm.nih.gov/pubmed/19399161. Accessed on November 15th 2019.

16. "A low-fat diet and/or strenuous exercise alters the ... - NCBI - NIH." https://www.ncbi.nlm.nih.gov/pubmed/12772189. Accessed on November 15th 2019.

17. "Intensive lifestyle changes may affect the ... - NCBI - NIH." https://www.ncbi.nlm.nih.gov/pubmed/16094059. Accessed on November 15th 2019.

18. "The power of nutrition as medicine. - NCBI." https://www.ncbi.nlm.nih.gov/pubmed/22561031. Accessed on November 15th 2019.

19. "The pediatric aspects of atherosclerosis. - NCBI." https://www.ncbi.nlm.nih.gov/pubmed/5346899. Accessed on November 15th 2019.

20. "Dietary approaches to prevent and treat hypertension ... - NCBI." https://www.ncbi.nlm.nih.gov/pubmed/16434724. Accessed on November 15th 2019.

21. "The role of Dietary Approaches to Stop Hypertension ... - NCBI." December 6th. 2018, https://www.ncbi.nlm.nih.gov/pubmed/22142820. Accessed on November 15th 2019.

22. "The total antioxidant content of more than 3100 foods ...
- NCBI." January 22nd 2010,
https://www.ncbi.nlm.nih.gov/pmc/articles/PMC2841576
/. Accessed on November 15th 2019.

23. "The key to halting progression of CKD might be in the
... - NCBI."
https://www.ncbi.nlm.nih.gov/pubmed/22170526.
Accessed on November 15th 2019.

24. "A new predictive equation for resting energy ... - NCBI
- NIH." https://www.ncbi.nlm.nih.gov/pubmed/2305711.
Accessed on November 15th 2019.

25. "Nutritious Wheat, whole grain, raw per 100 grams."
http://www.foodnutritiontable.com/nutritions/nutrient/?i
d=476. Accessed on November 15th 2019.

26. "Obesity and the development of type 2 diabetes: the ... -
NCBI." July 16th. 2010,
https://www.ncbi.nlm.nih.gov/pmc/articles/PMC3047970
/. Accessed on November 15th 2019.

27. "The Role of Body Fat and Fat Distribution in ... -
NCBI." May 12th 2016,
https://www.ncbi.nlm.nih.gov/pmc/articles/PMC4865112
/. Accessed on November 15th 2019.

28. "Atherosclerosis: Process, Indicators, Risk ...."
https://www.ncbi.nlm.nih.gov/pmc/articles/PMC4258672
/. Accessed on November 15th 2019.

29. "Peanuts as functional food: a review - NCBI." September
19th 2015,
https://www.ncbi.nlm.nih.gov/pmc/articles/PMC4711439
/. Accessed on November 15th 2019.

30. "Dietary Guidelines for Americans | HHS.gov." https://www.hhs.gov/fitness/eat-healthy/dietary-guidelines-for-americans/index.html. Accessed on November 15th 2019.

31. "Health Benefits of Fruits and Vegetables ...." July 6th 2012, https://www.ncbi.nlm.nih.gov/pmc/articles/PMC3649719/. Accessed on November 15th 2019.

32. "The human body and water | Otsuka Pharmaceutical Co., Ltd.." https://www.otsuka.co.jp/en/nutraceutical/about/rehydration/water/body-fluid/. Accessed on November 15th 2019.

33. "How much water should you drink? - Harvard Health." July 18th 2018, https://www.health.harvard.edu/staying-healthy/how-much-water-should-you-drink. Accessed on November 15th 2019.

34. "Dietary protein intake and human health - (RSC) Publishing." https://pubs.rsc.org/en/content/articlelanding/2016/fo/c5fo01530h. Accessed on November 15th 2019.

35. "Diets high in meat, eggs and dairy could be as harmful to ...." March 5th 2014, https://www.theguardian.com/science/2014/mar/04/animal-protein-diets-smoking-meat-eggs-dairy. Accessed on November 15th 2019.

36. "Low protein intake is associated with a major ... - NCBI - NIH." March 4th 2014, https://www.ncbi.nlm.nih.gov/pubmed/24606898. Accessed on November 15th 2019.

37. "The Fast Diet Review: What to Expect - WebMD."
March 4th 2019, https://www.webmd.com/diet/a-z/fast-diet-review. Accessed on November 15th 2019.

38. "Dr John Tilden – Whole Food Plant Based Diet." July 25th 2018, https://www.wholefoodplantbaseddiet.com/tag/dr-john-tilden/. Accessed on November 15th 2019.

39. "The Vegetarian Resource Group (VRG) | DR. JOHN HARVEY ...." https://www.vrg.org/history/DrJohnHarveyKellogg.htm. Accessed on November 15th 2019.

40. "Bernarr McFadden's Physical Culture Cookbook – Physical ...." June 28th 2016, https://physicalculturestudy.com/2016/06/28/bernarr-mcfaddens-physical-culture-cookbook/. Accessed on November 15th 2019.

41. "St. Louis Estes | Revolvy." https://www.revolvy.com/page/St.-Louis-Estes. Accessed on November 15th 2019.

42. "Naturopathic Medicine: What It Is, Benefits, Risks - WebMD." March 15th 2019, https://www.webmd.com/balance/guide/what-is-naturopathic-medicine. Accessed on November 15th2019.

43. "Henry Lindlahr - ND Health Facts." August 3rd 2012, http://www.ndhealthfacts.org/wiki/Henry_Lindlahr. Accessed on November 15th 2019.

44. "stuffy nose | vegan food | mucusless diet pdf | mucusless diet ...." February 17th 2017,

https://www.mucusfreelife.com/about/what-is-the-mucusless-diet/. Accessed on November 15th 2019.

45. "Angina and vegan diet. - NCBI." https://www.ncbi.nlm.nih.gov/pubmed/860681. Accessed on November 15th 2019.

46. "Cancer incidence in vegetarians: results from the ... - NCBI." March 11th 2009, https://www.ncbi.nlm.nih.gov/pubmed/19279082. Accessed on November 15th 2019.

47. "Meat and cheese may be as bad for you as smoking - USC ...." March 4th 2014, https://pressroom.usc.edu/meat-and-cheese-may-be-as-bad-for-you-as-smoking/. Accessed on November 15th 2019.

48. "High-carbohydrate, high-fiber diets for insulin-treated ... - NCBI." https://www.ncbi.nlm.nih.gov/pubmed/495550. Accessed on November 15th 2019.

49. "Usefulness of vegetarian and vegan diets for treating ... - NCBI." https://www.ncbi.nlm.nih.gov/pubmed/20425575. Accessed on November 15th 2019.

50. "Associations of diet with albuminuria and kidney ... - NCBI - NIH." March 18th 2010, https://www.ncbi.nlm.nih.gov/pubmed/20299364. Accessed on November 15th 2019.

51. "Comparison of a vegetable-based (soya) and an ... - NCBI." https://www.ncbi.nlm.nih.gov/pubmed/9647497. Accessed on November 15th 2019.

52. "Low blood pressure in vegetarians: effects of ... - NCBI - NIH." https://www.ncbi.nlm.nih.gov/pubmed/3414588. Accessed on November 15th 2019.

53. "Beyond meatless, the health effects of vegan ... - NCBI - NIH." May 27th 2014, https://www.ncbi.nlm.nih.gov/pubmed/24871675. Accessed on November 15th 2019.

54. "The relation of protein foods to hypertension. - NCBI." https://www.ncbi.nlm.nih.gov/pubmed/18739909. Accessed on November 15th 2019.

55. "Blood pressure in the African native. - The Lancet." https://www.thelancet.com/journals/lancet/article/PIIS0140-6736(00)49248-2/fulltext. Accessed on November 15th 2019.

56. "PubMed - NCBI." https://www.ncbi.nlm.nih.gov/pubmed/214199. Accessed on November 15th 2019.

57. "Blood Pressure Amongst Aboriginal Ethnic ... - The Lancet." https://www.thelancet.com/journals/lancet/article/PIIS0140-6736(00)86708-2/fulltext. Accessed on November 15th 2019.

58. "Health benefits of physical activity: the ...." March 14th 2006, https://www.ncbi.nlm.nih.gov/pmc/articles/PMC1402378/. Accessed on November 15th 2019.

59. "Happier People Live More Active Lives: Using ... - NCBI." January 4th 2017,

https://www.ncbi.nlm.nih.gov/pmc/articles/PMC5213770/. Accessed on November 15th 2019.

60. "Happiness & Health: The Biological Factors ... - NCBI." https://www.ncbi.nlm.nih.gov/pmc/articles/PMC4449495/. Accessed on November 15th 2019.

61. "Exercise: How much do I need every day? - Mayo Clinic." https://www.mayoclinic.org/healthy-lifestyle/fitness/expert-answers/exercise/faq-20057916. Accessed on November 15th 2019.

62. "No level of alcohol consumption improves health – The Lancet." https://www.thelancet.com/article/S0140-6736(18)31571-X/fulltext. Accessed on November 15th 2019.

63. "CAGE Questionnaire." http://nationalpaincentre.mcmaster.ca/documents/cage_questionnaire.pdf. Accessed on November 15th 2019.

64. "Tobacco smoking: Health impact, prevalence ... - NCBI." May 28th 2017, https://www.ncbi.nlm.nih.gov/pmc/articles/PMC5490618/. Accessed on November 15th 2019.

65. "Clinical Effects of Cigarette Smoking - NCBI - NIH." September 28th 2017, https://www.ncbi.nlm.nih.gov/pmc/articles/PMC5664648/. Accessed on November 15th 2019.

66. "Effectiveness of Hypnosis Techniques to Quit Smoking ...." September 28th 2018, https://ascopubs.org/doi/abs/10.1200/jgo.18.80200. Accessed on November 15th 2019.

67. "The relationship between physical and mental health: A ...."
    https://www.sciencedirect.com/science/article/pii/S02779
    53617306639. Accessed on November 15th 2019.

68. "STRESS AND HEALTH: Psychological ... - NCBI -
    NIH."
    https://www.ncbi.nlm.nih.gov/pmc/articles/PMC2568977
    /. Accessed on November 15th 2019.

69. "The impact of stress on body function: A ...." July 21st
    2017,
    https://www.ncbi.nlm.nih.gov/pmc/articles/PMC5579396
    /. Accessed on November 15th 2019.

70. "Short- and long-term health consequences of sleep ... -
    NCBI." May 19th 2017,
    https://www.ncbi.nlm.nih.gov/pmc/articles/PMC5449130
    /. Accessed on November 15th 2019.

71. "Making health habitual: the psychology of 'habit ... -
    NCBI."
    https://www.ncbi.nlm.nih.gov/pmc/articles/PMC3505409
    /. Accessed on November 15th 2019.